Table of Contents

Table of Contents

Introduction

What is Electromedicine?

History of Electromedicine

Call to Action

Introduction

Bioelectric Systems

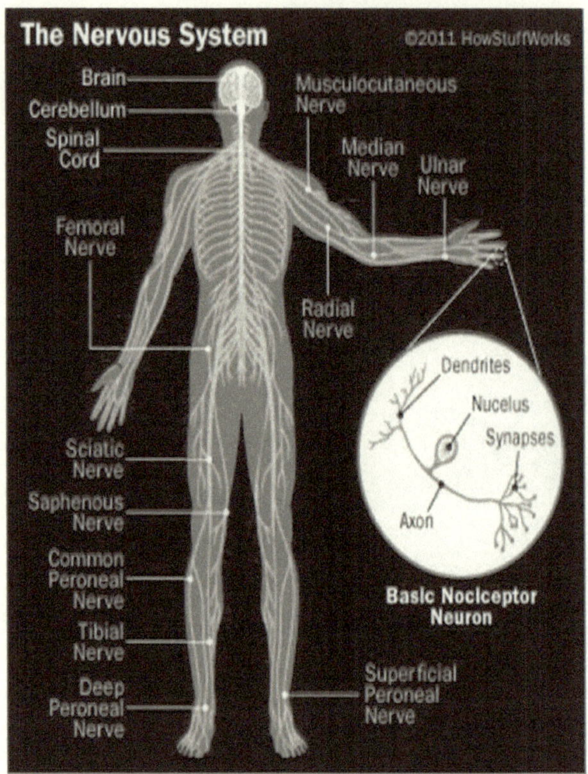

Well, what is this about? Most of us think of medicine, the practice of medicine, as needles, drugs, and surgery. Those three things, that's all we need. We need to become addicted to drugs, we need to have marks on our skin from needles and scars from the surgery that is performed to take care of the problems we have. That's pretty much what we're looking at, right? This is called allopathic medicine. It's standard medicine. That's what's practiced in America, unlike Europe, Russia, or Canada, where they're a bit more progressive. I'm going to talk about the old/new field of electromedicine. I say old/new because whenever I explain it to people, they say, "Why haven't I heard about this before? It's new, isn't it?"

Yes it's new, since it was invented in 1979 in America and sold worldwide, electromedicine started at **Medtronic** the way it's practiced today in

America. At Medtronic, where I worked in 1979, we invented, designed, and put out to the world the first **TENS unit**. It was a small electrical device the size of a packet of cigarettes with wires and electrodes which, when attached to the body in an area of pain, stopped the pain signal. I was one of the inventors of this device. Medtronic sold 56 million of them from 1981- 1984.

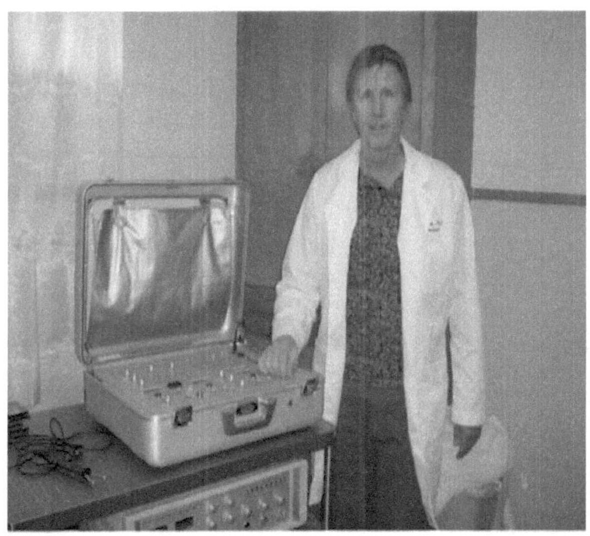

Other companies I've worked for since then have sold millions more, yet I still keep getting asked the question, Why is this so new and why haven't I heard of it before? It's because it's suppressed. There's a better way to do things than needles, drugs, pills, pharmaceuticals, and surgery.

The old/new field of electromedicine kind of goes like this: It is a field of medicine wherein equipment is designed which interacts with the body electronically. The human body is an **electro-chemical** system. It operates on an electric circuit. The body is an electric circuit. These circuits, the nodes of these circuits, are cells. The body is full of billions of cells. Each cell is an electrical piece. It has a positive and a negative charge. They're called ions and they circle the cell. They're in the aqueous fluid around the cell and they're positively charged, negatively charged, neutrally charged, depending on the function of the cell.

Our bodies are made up of billions of them. Inside of each cell is a battery, just like the stuff we plug in our ears and plug everywhere else and use. The battery is called the mitochondria. The **mitochondria** is the cell energy-producing battery of the cell function. They are the activators. Outside of it is the substance that carries the cell and is **charged positively or negatively**. The body is made up of muscles and nerves and other soft tissue. This soft tissue is fed, nourished, and grows by the production of **protein**, which is produced by the transfer of **ions** across the cells, which multiply, producing more protein, converting biochemicals, stimulating the sodium potassium pump in the body. All biochemistry, electrochemistry, this is how the body works. Little tiny engines, the cells, keep reproducing, keep functioning, keep pushing the system and the organs to work. To repair them, to grow them, to replace them constantly.

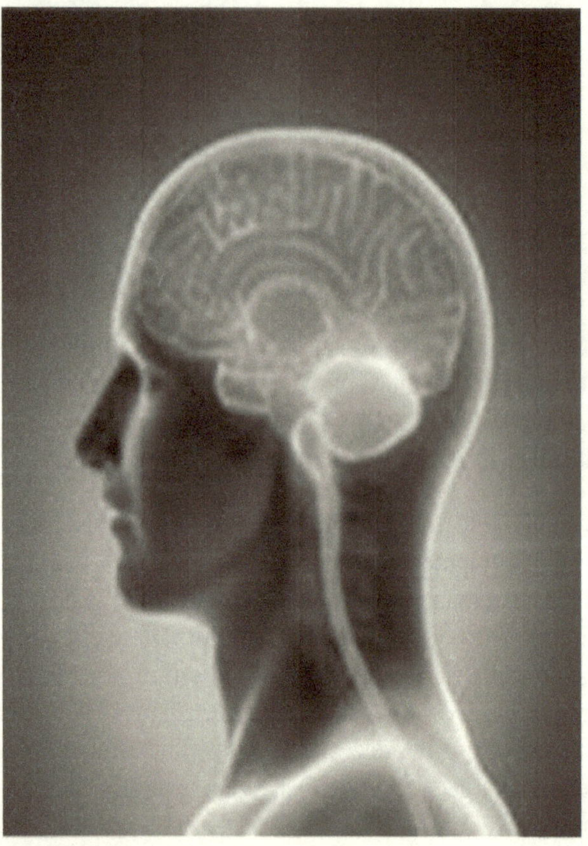

The human body replaces itself in its entirety every six months. What happens is that you have something wrong with your body, if you treat it right, if you reprogram it, the body will repair itself in six months and rid itself of the memory of the old injury or disease. That is pretty much the formula for healthy, functioning cell function. What happens when we have an injury? What happens is that all of this gets changed. The polarity in the cells change, the positive and the negative ions will multiply in one direction or the other, the body becomes out of balance. Electrochemically out of balance. This results in an injury, pain, chronicity, and destruction of the tissue. The injury itself, when it happens and the moment it happens, produces what is called a current of injury.

The current of injury is like a virus. Say you are in a football game and you get hurt, crashed into, your rotator cuff becomes injured, damaged, traumatized, the current of injury immediately starts, and then what once was something the size of your finger, starts growing. If you let it go several hours, overnight, the next day, a few days later, by the time you get to the doctor it's now what started this size at minute one is this size a day or two later because the virus grew, the current of injury grew.

All the cells in the injury then became damaged, malfunctioning, which caused the body's prehistoric method of protection: inflammation, closing the blood supply to the tissue and basically walling off and breaking down the healing process. The healing process needs to occur in order for the injury to get well and go away but what happens is it goes in the reverse to protect itself. So what we do in electromedicine is to put a signal into the body to change that, to correct each and every cell so they're functioning normally and in a healthy manner, to reproduce and to correct themselves, which then will lead to increasing blood supply, reduction of edema, swelling, inflammation. **Returning the body back to its normal state.**

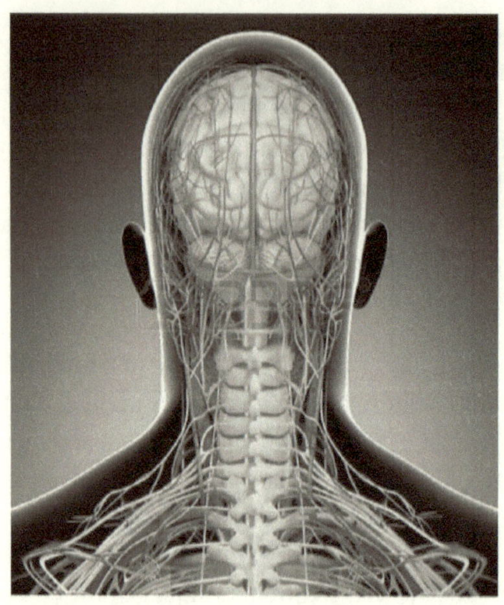

There are two kinds of injuries. There's the acute stage, where it just happened and the current of injury has just occurred and it's growing, and there's the chronic stage where the injury occurred a month or two ago, a few years ago, and the injury stayed with the body, stayed with the memory system of the cell. The cells have a memory. They each remember the way it was so they reproduce the way it was to be the way it will be, which is the way it was. So the cell memory carries forward through the years. This is called a **chronic state of injury.**

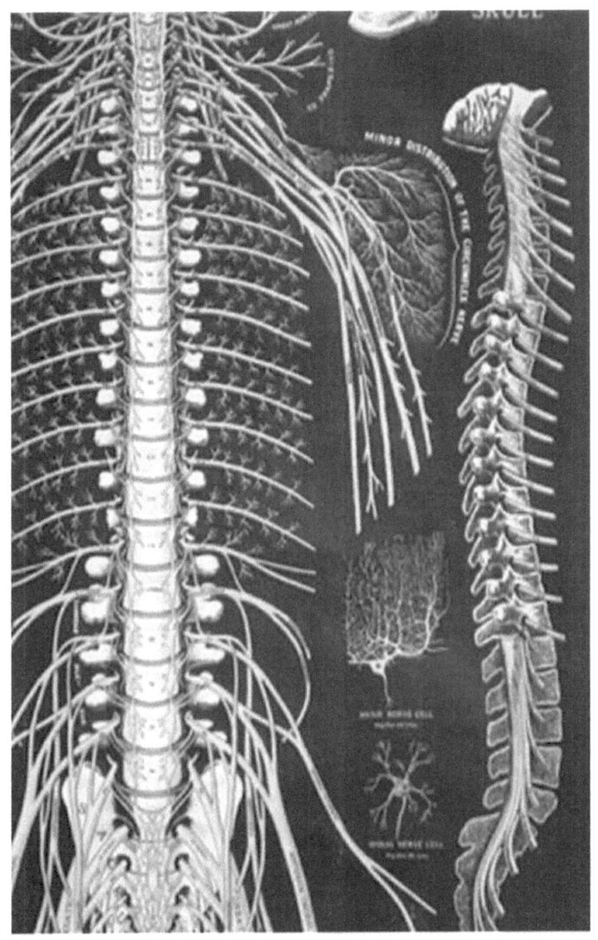

To break the chronic state of injury, the trauma, the memory in the cell, we reprogram the cell with a computer. I have designed computers for 30 years that do this. They are sold worldwide and used in clinical practice. Why haven't I heard of this before? Well, watch. Go somewhere, go to physical therapists, go to chiropractors. Chiropractors, by the way, I have found to be the biggest risk-takers in many ways in the field of electro medicine. The chiropractors have been the ones who primarily took this equipment and used it in their practices because they have the training to do this. They took this and guess what? Their practices improved and they got better and they had better results.

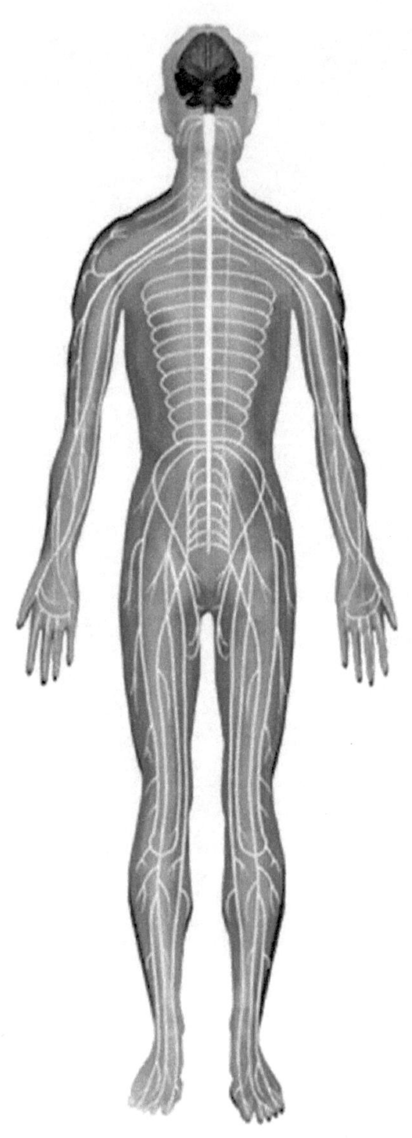

Chiropractors, from a structural point of view and **electrotherapy** from a biochemical/muscle/soft tissue point of view, can pretty well wrap up the problems that people have. Accurately diagnose them and repair them because an injury will cause a structural damage and soft tissue damage, so if we put the spinal column in the right alignment and then we treat the tissue and repair it, and we find we're able to accomplish a great deal this way.

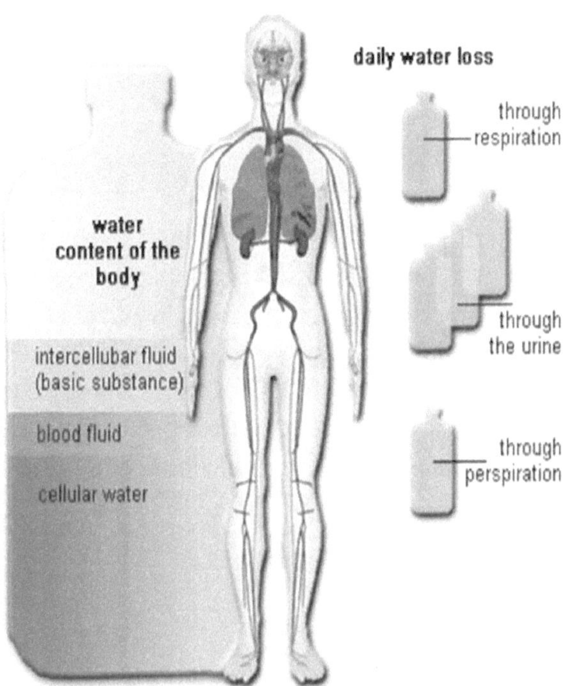

The computers we have designed to do this, interface with the human body in the sense of you hardly feel it, they're hooked up to you, the injury is treated with handheld probes, electrodes, etc., attached to the body, run a few minutes a current into the body, and right at that moment, they are repaired, repaired instantly. A traumatic injury occurring in the moment, can be stopped and repaired. I'm going to give you a live example of that. The injury, in essence, in my work with athletic teams including the Dallas Cowboys and other high school and college teams, we have found that a player that is injured—let's say an offensive lineman is injured, he comes off the field, he's treated, and it only takes five or six minutes to do it, he goes in the next set of downs, uninjured because the injury was erased. That's very possible; we do it all the time. In order to do this, we use different kinds of equipment.

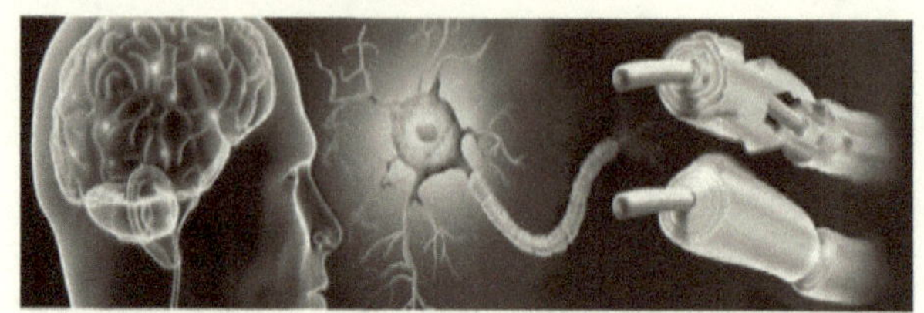

One of the first projects I was involved in was **The Electro-Accuscope**, which is one of the first micro-current devices—micro-current, millionths of an amp, not a car battery, not jumper cables, a millionth of an amp. The average treatment current of the Electro-Accuscope, which reads the tissue, puts back a signal to correct what it reads. It's called a positive feedback loop. The average is somewhere in the neighborhood of half a Hertz and approximately 80-300 micro amps. That's 300 millionths of one amp. Very small. You don't feel it.

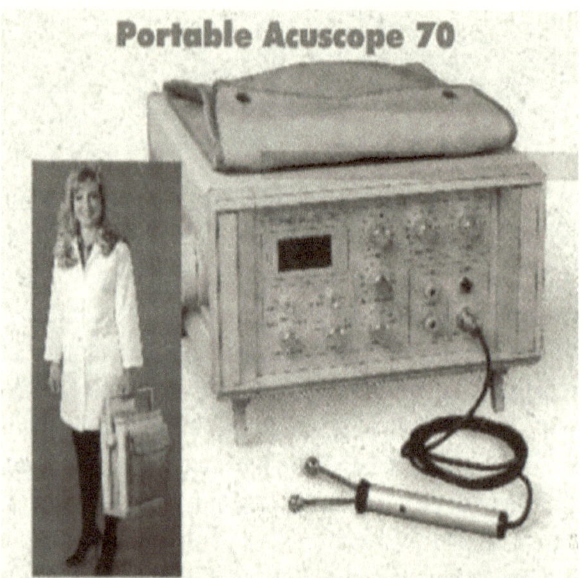

I was on the design team for the **Myomatic** in 1980; we developed this device and it's sold and used all over the country. It cost $3,000 and was used in practices all over the country to repair injuries. Basically how it works is that the machine is turned on, the settings are adjusted for the output that you want, what kind of injury you want to repair, what depth you want to go, etc.

Then wherever the injury is, it is treated here for 15 seconds, here for 15 seconds, here, here, let's say around the rotator cuff. So you have a treatment time of maybe 10 minutes for an injury. If it's an acute injury that just happened that day or the day before, all you need is maybe one or two treatments and you're done! It's fixed. You didn't have to go to the hospital, go to the doctor, physical therapy, take time off work, whatever, none of it. It's done.

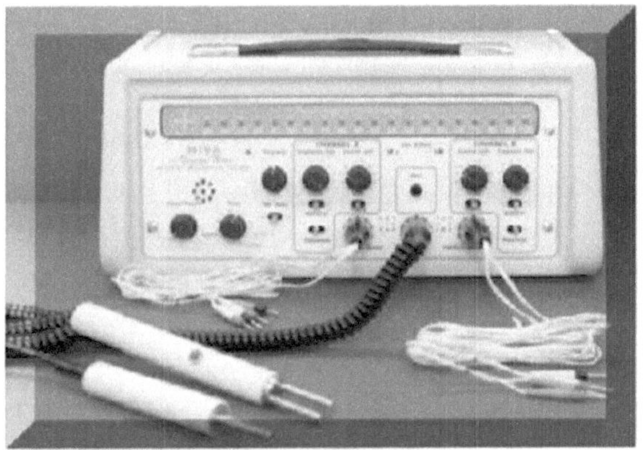

This is how this device works. It goes into the body, it reads the problem, and corrects it automatically. There's a lot of training that goes into teaching somebody how to use this. I have trained people myself, there are trainers that will train therapists how to use it, it's in the protocol where to treat, how to treat, how to have a sense about how to work with the human body. We have two probes; one is held in one hand and has a button on it. And you go here and you read the body until you find the point of injury. The machine will open up and will tell you…(buzzing noise)…that's a perfect circuit there. Now what that says is that there's a full connection so that you would treat and you push the button. Now the Accuscope is the same principle.

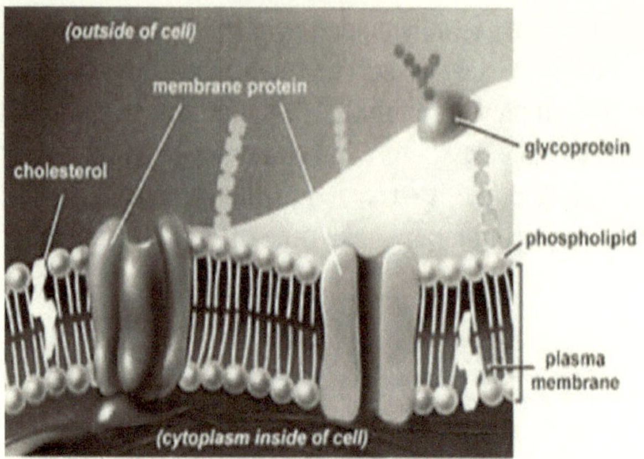

The computers, they are computers, are put in touch with the human body, with the injury, and then they are put to work to repair it and they do it immediately. Now the average is like this—if it's an acute injury, it's done in one, maybe two treatments, if it's a chronic injury, like a year or longer, it may take six, maybe nine treatments, and then the injury is repaired.

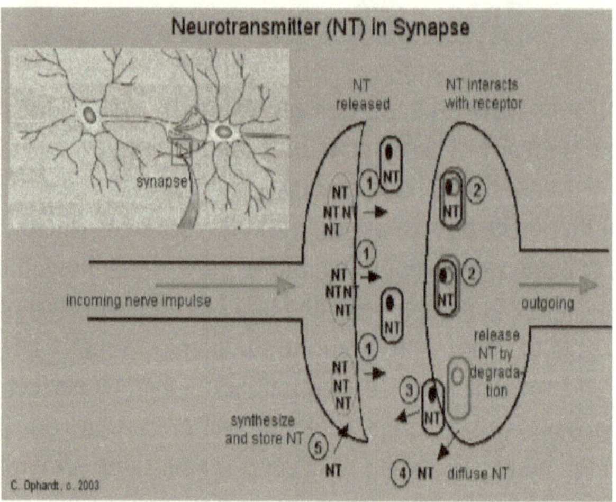

The next step in this whole progression is now getting smaller. So we have really big thing here, really big show, we have a smaller big show, and now what we're coming to is a smaller show. Well it's in here now. How does this work? Well, it works this way. We have this little unit and we have this probe, and all we do to treat a patient is I hold this, I find it, this reads the body, finds the injury, and repairs it. That's what we do. We literally find the injury, stop the pain, and return the body back to normal in a few minutes.

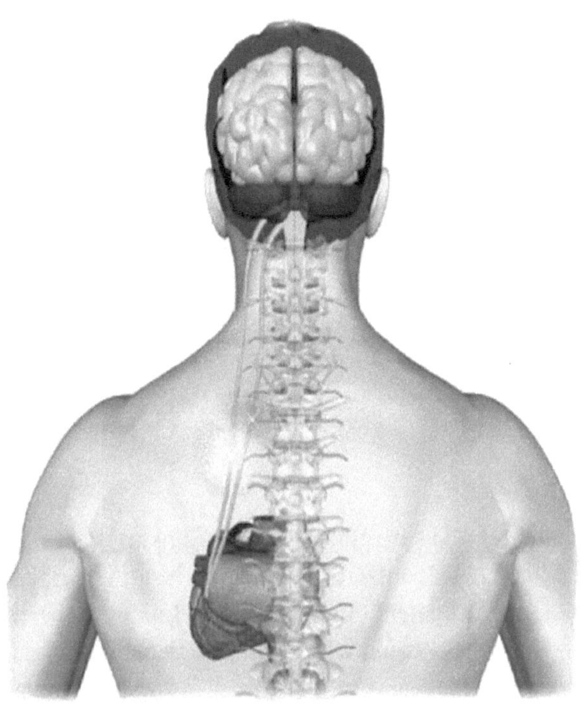

I would like to tell you a couple of things about this kind of technology; some of the patients that I see and some of the injuries and disorders that I treat. They include whiplash injuries, lumbar strains, low back injuries, chronic low back pain, rotator cuff injuries, trigeminal neuralgia which is severe pain of the face.

For example, I had a patient this year that came in with 20 years of trigeminal neuralgia. 18 years of unceasing chronic, severe pain in the right side of his face. When he came in to see me, his face was askew, it was not symmetrical. His eye drooped, his lip drooped, he didn't look right. I treated him, repaired him, stopped the pain, and reconfigured his face so he left with no pain, no trigeminal neuralgia, and his face was symmetrical. That's one thing I do with this equipment.

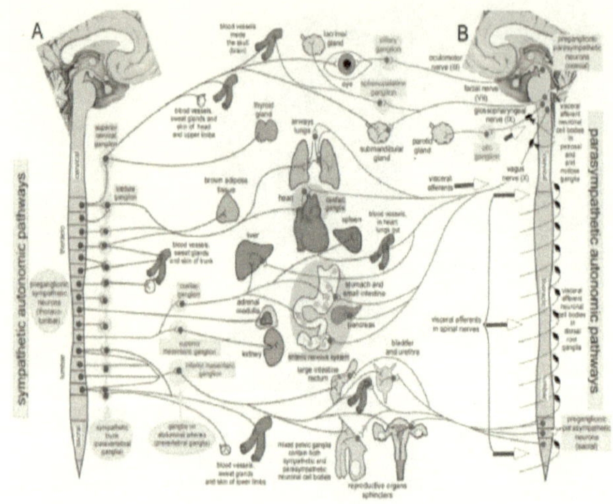

Other treatments that we do are athletic injuries, ankles, knees. I tore my medial cruciate ligament a couple of years ago. I heard it tear, I swear I did, it was ugly. I used this equipment to repair myself. I did it in two days. I repaired my leg such that I could walk again. I was badly injured. I played tennis two weeks after the tear. I'm not slow. I'm very fast and aggressive.

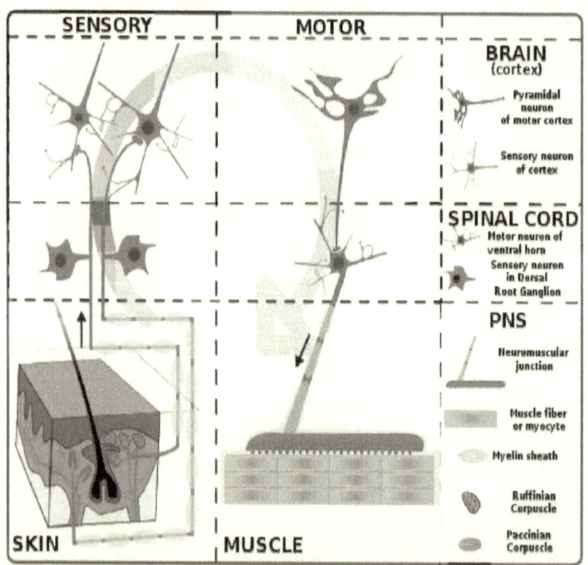

The thing is, this stuff works. I'll call it **"new" medicine**. I've only been in it 30 years; I guess it's still new. It does work. We can do pretty much miracle kind of medicine. Some of the kinds of injuries I treat include carpel tunnel syndrome, peripheral neuralgia, paralysis, lack of sensation, parenthetic injuries, strains, sprains, tears, rotator cuff injuries, anterior cruciate ligament tears, strains. I can repair the tissue at the cellular level by reprogramming it with this equipment.

This is pretty much what I do. I call myself a television repair man for the human body. Bring in your set, I'll attach my tools and fix it. What we can do then, is electronically change the signal, so the signal does not say hurt, it says '**NORMAL**'. So we can do this electronically and we've been doing it for years

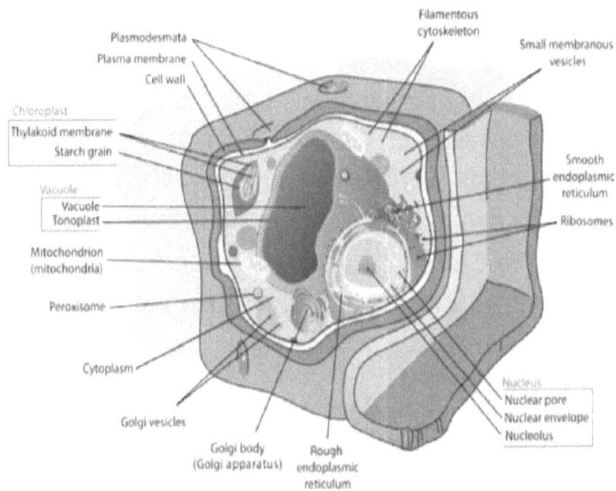

I have been thinking about how I explain to clients what is happening in their body when soft tissue is injured. One way I describe a new or fresh soft tissue injury is like a pebble thrown into the middle of a still lake. Think about it - skipping pebbles at the lake. "See" what happens when it "plops". An injury is just like this. It often starts as just a very tiny circle. As the minutes and hours pass an injury grows like the circles in the lake from the initial "plop" of the tossed pebble.

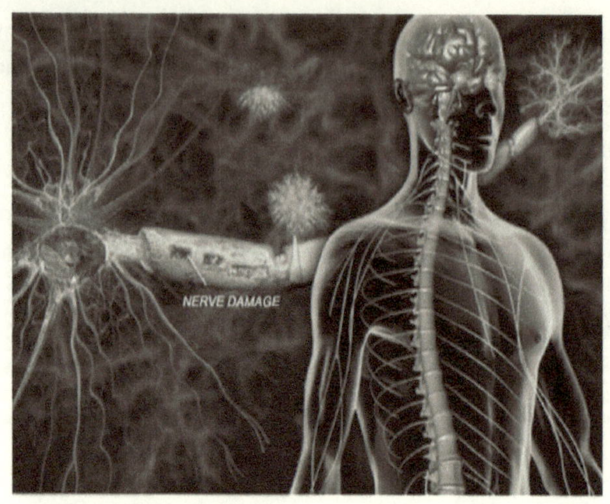

Injuries grow immediately through involvement of cell after cell after nerve, muscle, and tendon or ligament fiber. **Biochemicals** gather about the injury to wall it off from the rest of the body, producing swelling and inflammation as a "warning" not to use the injured part. This process is not necessary today as we, unlike the caveman, have no need to keep fighting, surviving, or using the injured appendage. Still the injury grows, involving more and more tissue. It rapidly swells and becomes painful.

What to Do?

If you have a **regenerative electrotherapy** device like a **SCENAR** you would treat yourself immediately. Yes, home units are available. I see the day when we will all have one in our home. They are not complicated to use and they are worth it over your lifetime. Actually my experience is that most people get their return on investment with one, maybe two injuries or issues. Better a SCENAR in your home than a bottle of pills given their side effect profiles.

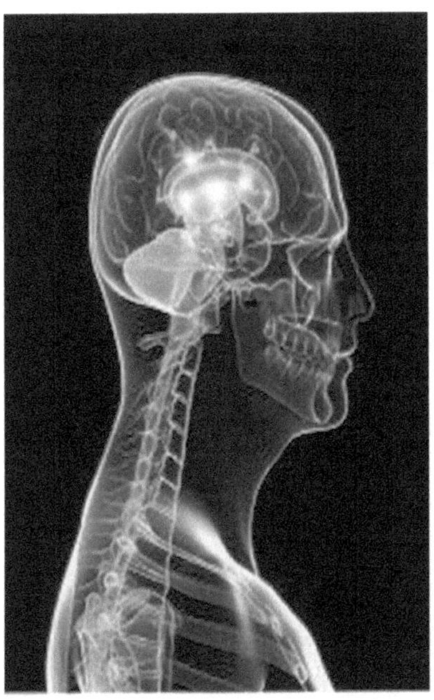

The sooner a regenerative electrotherapy modality like SCENAR is applied the sooner an injury can be repaired. It could be as soon as overnight if applied the same day as the injury. Really.

If you don't have a SCENAR

So you don't have your own SCENAR yet. Well, this is the injury that might make you say "now". What you need to do is immediately, within minutes, sit or lie down and apply ice to try to stop the progression of the injury. Use ice for 20 minutes several times during the day of the injury. Taking an **anti-inflammatory** several times the first couple of days of the injury can also be useful. I suggest fish oil. Rest the injury!

What is Electromedicine?

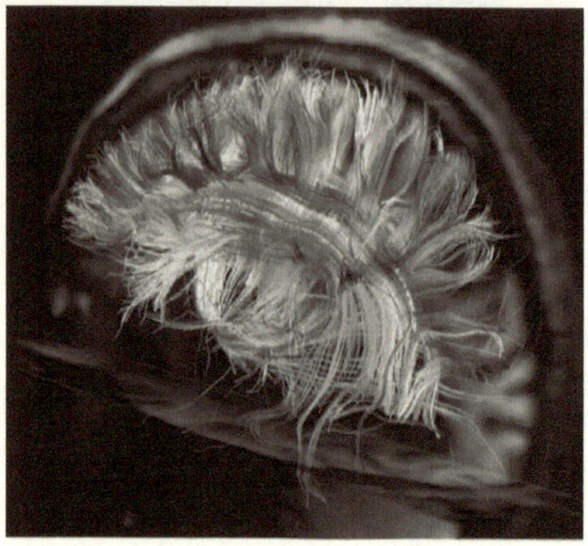

Basic research on cells in culture, animals, and clinical studies led to specific information on the frequency, amplitude, orientation, and exposure characteristics required to activate specific processes in specific cells. As a result, we now have a sophisticated understanding of the mechanism of action of **bioelectromagnetic therapies**—with a detailed picture of the cascade of reactions taking place from the cell surface to the cytoplasm and on to the nucleus and genes—where selective effects on transcription and translation have been documented.

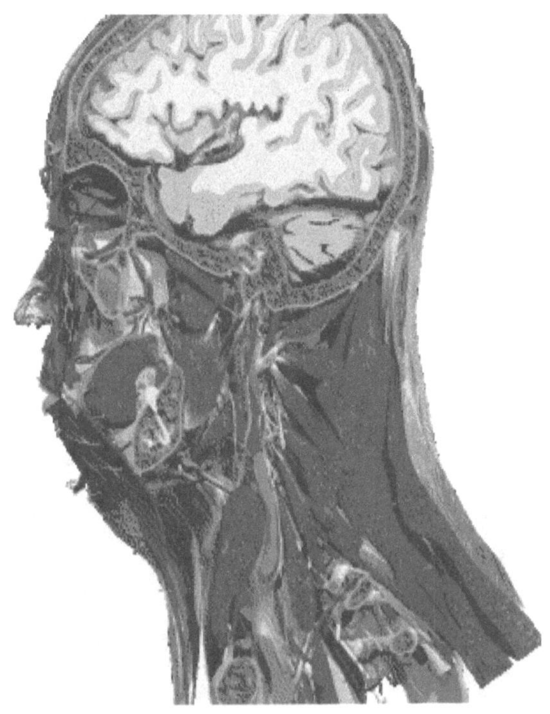

A single antigen, hormone, pheromone, growth factor, smell or taste or neurotransmitter molecule, or a single photon of electromagnetic energy can produce a cascade of intracellular signals that initiate, accelerate, or inhibit biological processes. This is possible because of enormous amplification. A single molecular event at the cell surface can trigger a huge influx of calcium ions, each of which can activate an enzyme.

The enzymes, in turn, act as catalysts, greatly accelerating biochemical processes. The enzymes are not consumed by these reactions and can therefore act repeatedly. Some of the reactions are sensitive to electromagnetic fields, some are not. Others have not yet been tested. Some frequencies enhance calcium entry, while others diminish it. Steps in the cascade involving free radical formation are likely targets of magnetic fields.

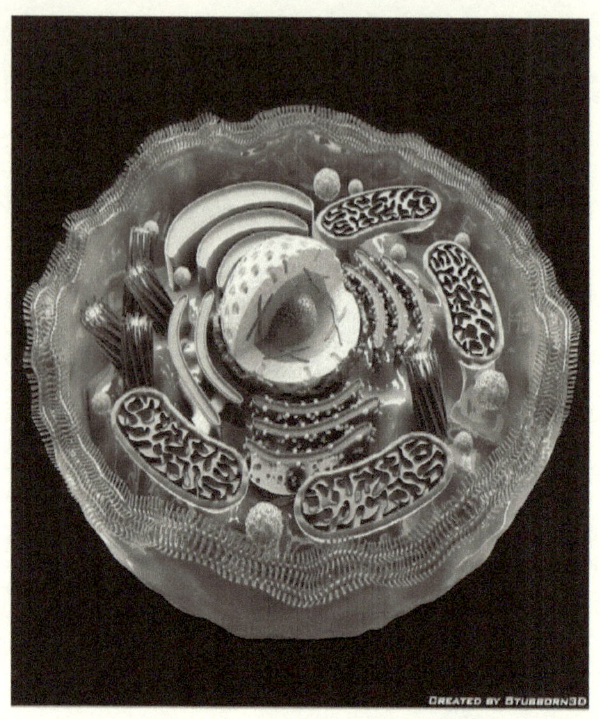

After decades of clinical success with the use of **PEMF** for bone, attention turned naturally to injuries of soft tissues, such as nerve, skin, muscle, and tendon and the pain associated with those injuries. Unlike the situation in the late 1800s, however, these applications are being developed with appropriate mechanistic understandings and clinical verification.

Siskin and Walker summarize the results with various soft tissues. **The following effects have been observed:**

Enhanced capillary formation

Decreased necrosis

Reduced swelling

Diminished pain

Faster functional recovery

Reduction in depth, area, and pain in skin wounds

Reduced muscle loss after ligament surgery

Increased tensile strength in ligaments

Acceleration of nerve regeneration and functional recovery.

Another crucial step in the revival of electrotherapeutics was the development of transcutaneous electrical nerve stimulation (TENS). In 1965, **Melzack and Wall** proposed the gate control theory of pain. A few years later, **C. Normal Shealy, M.D,** a neurosurgeon who had been routinely implanting dorsal column stimulators (**DCS**) that he had developed to control pain, discovered that the electric signals could be introduced from the skin surface, providing pain control without the risks of surgery. After a lengthy and difficult interaction with the FDA, the TENS unit was recognized as safe and effective, and there are now more than 100 different FDA approved devices in this category, with some 250,000 **TENS** units prescribed annually in the United States alone.

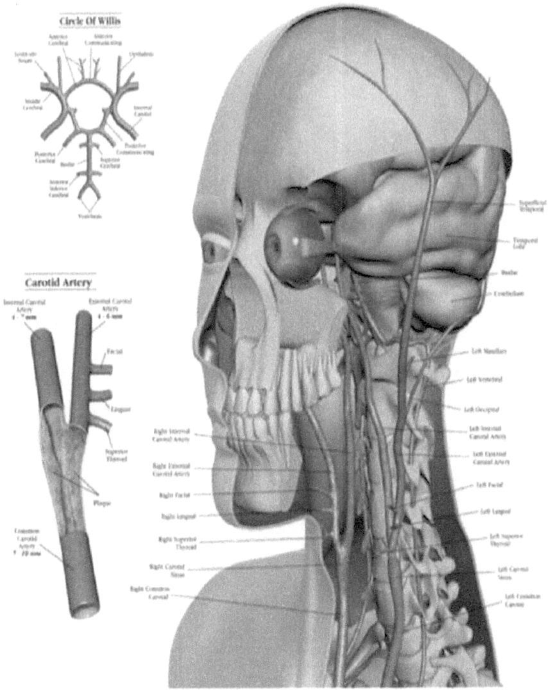

Fluid systems of the body, including the circulatory system and extracellular fluids of various kinds, act as virtual antennas for externally applied fields. These fluids are highly conductive because they contain electrically charged ions, predominantly sodium, potassium, and chloride. More subtle but perhaps far more significant effects occur because the proteins and other molecules comprising the tissues are semiconductors.

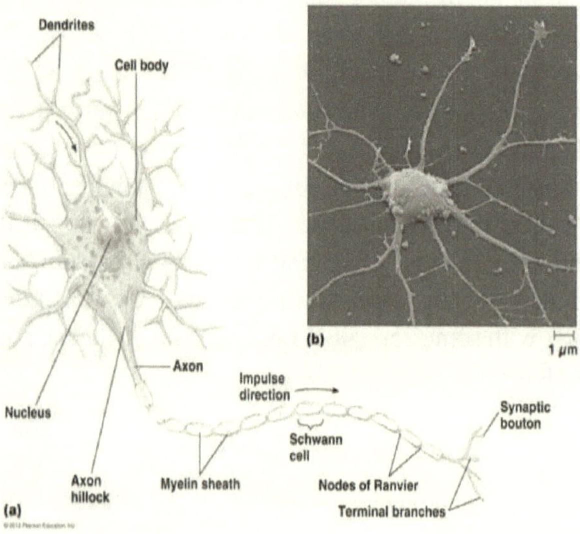

Mention has been made of the early development of biological electronics and applications of solid-state physics to living systems. We now know that the human body is composed of an interconnected semiconductor fibrous matrix that extends into its every nook and cranny. Macroscopically, this system consists of the connective tissues that form bones, tendons, fascia, cartilage, and ligaments and that also form the matrix of all **organs** and **glands**. All of the great systems of the body, the musculature, vasculature, nervous system, digestive tract, integument, and lymphatics are composed of connective tissue that gives them their characteristic form and physical properties. Cell biologists have now discerned how this continuous fibrous system connects with cell surfaces and cell interiors via transmembrane proteins such as the integrins.

The Cell

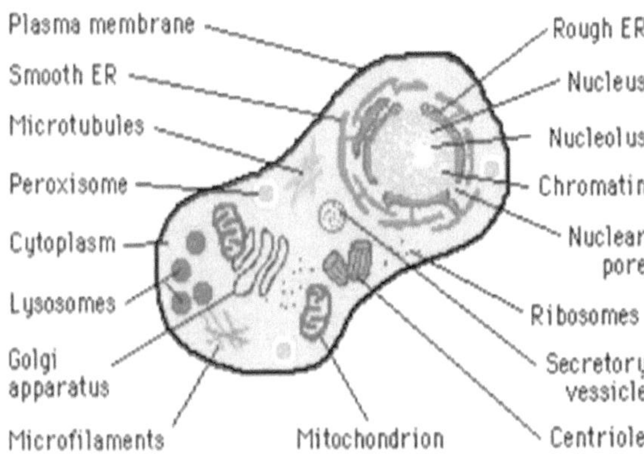

The figure below details the **extracellular matrix** and its continuity with the cytoskeleton and nuclear matrix. It is significant that all components of this continuous system are liquid crystalline semiconductors, features that confer a variety of interesting properties to the material substance of the body. Future developments in **bioelectromagnetics** will undoubtedly emerge from the study of the living body as an integrated electronic and protonic circuit.

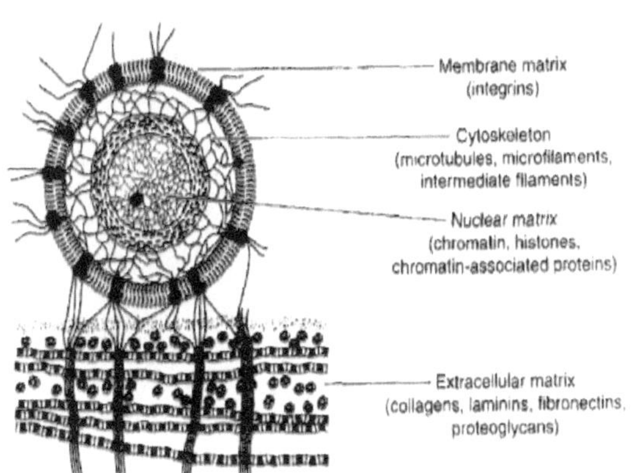

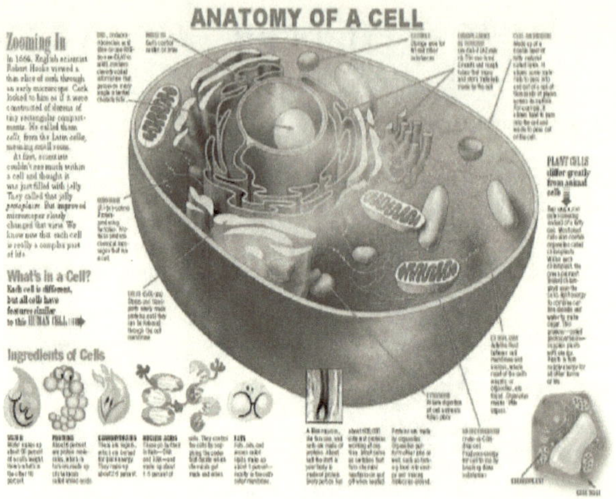

While skepticism remains, modern science has essentially resolved the issues that have surrounded **bioelectromagnetics** and that have led to so much bitter controversy in the past. This progress is vitally important for the future evolution of medicine. The energetic perspective has, perhaps more than any other, been blinded by confusion and debate, significantly slowing medical progress. The confusion and controversy have benefited the very profitable pharmaceutical approach, which has dominated modern medicine in spite of its enormous costs and debilitating side effects. By following the energetic thread that runs through all therapies we are opening up a discussion that is having a dramatic impact on the future of medicine.

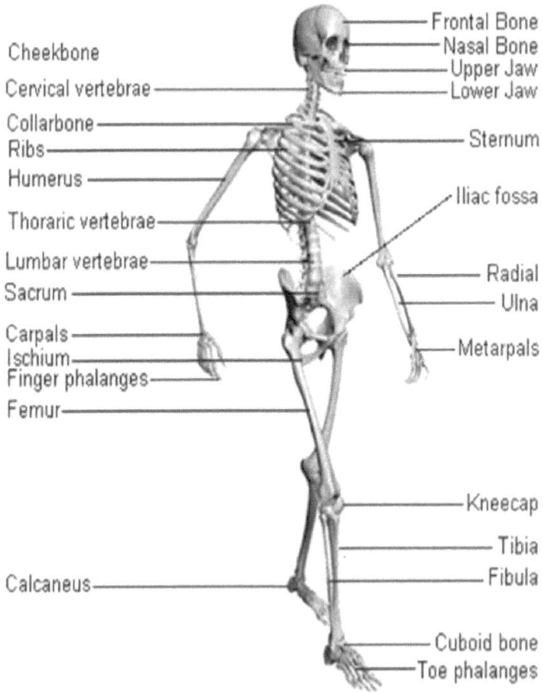

Bioelectromagnetics offers a tremendous opportunity to create a new and more effective kind of medicine with very specific effects and virtually no toxic side effects. Inordinately complex and arbitrary regulatory hurdles are hindering the emergence of this field, and another way of separating the wheat from the chaff is definitely needed if we are to survive the current crisis in health care and experience the full potential **bioelectromagnetic medicine** has to offer. For we are living in a time when the health care system is in severe crisis due to high costs, and we are experiencing several epidemics simultaneously, e.g., cancer and AIDS and chronic exposure to deadly toxins such as pesticides of all kinds and aspartame and related sugar substitutes.

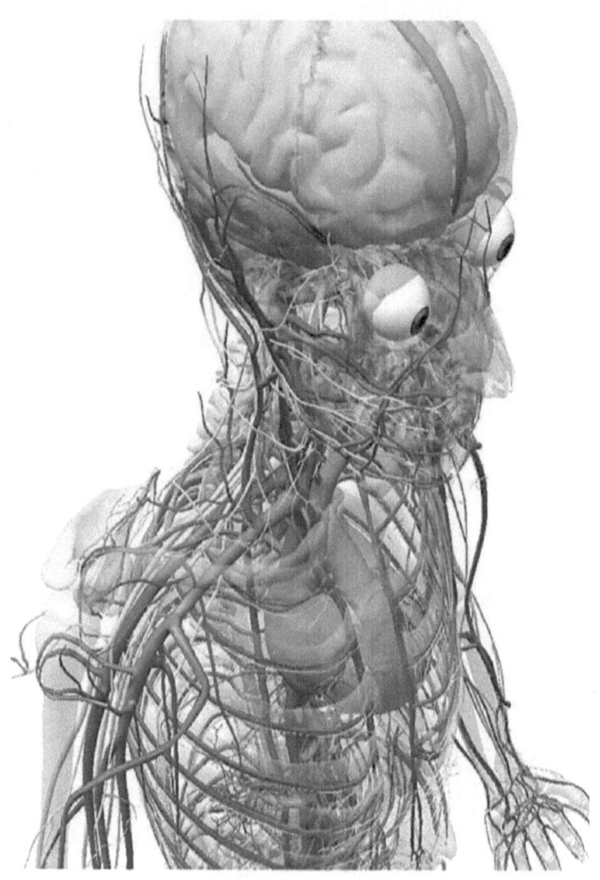

Energetic phenomena serve as a focal point for discussing both causes and treatments in new and productive ways. Many of the complementary therapies have energetic concepts as part of their theoretical base, and these methods not only are becoming quite popular, but also show promise for treating the chronic patient whose problems are the most costly in terms of suffering and in terms of health-care dollars, and whose lingering difficulties often frustrate the conventional physician.

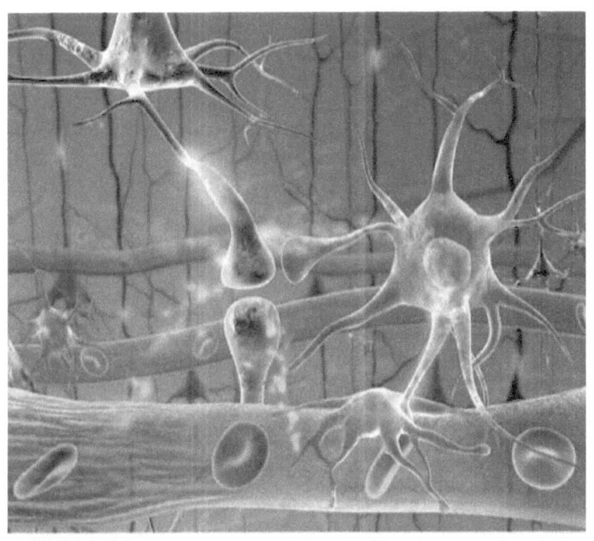

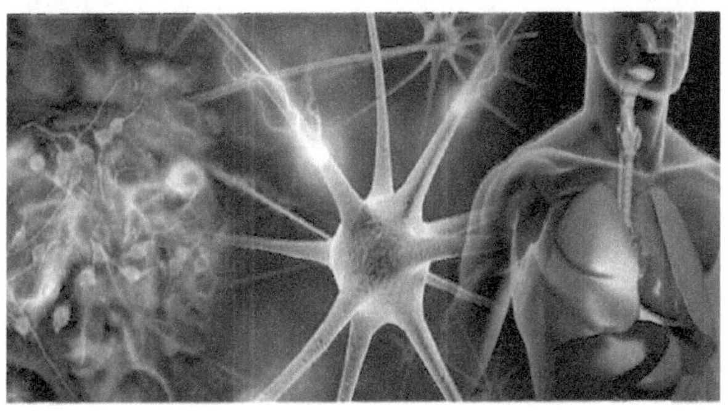

History of Electromedicine

This whole system started a long time ago. We can make reference to Royal Rife in 1935 and his landmark work in finding cures for cancer and many other diseases by changing the electrochemical function of cells, and reading the cells and changing their electrochemical properties.

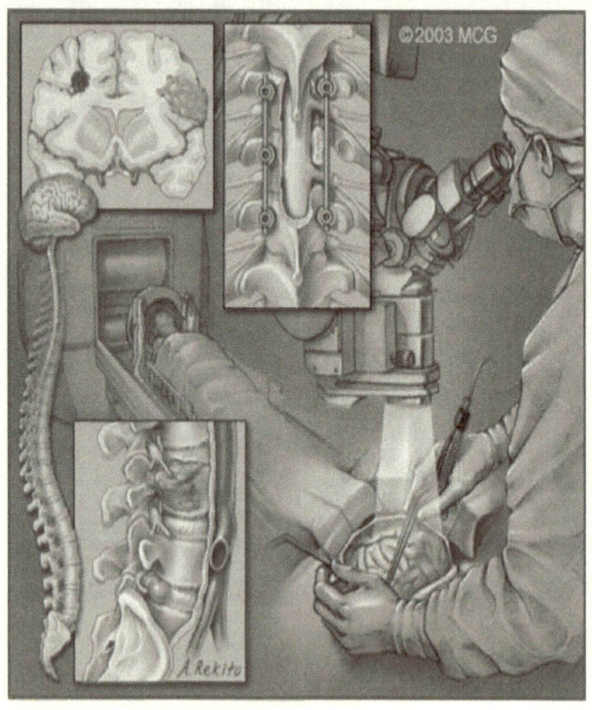

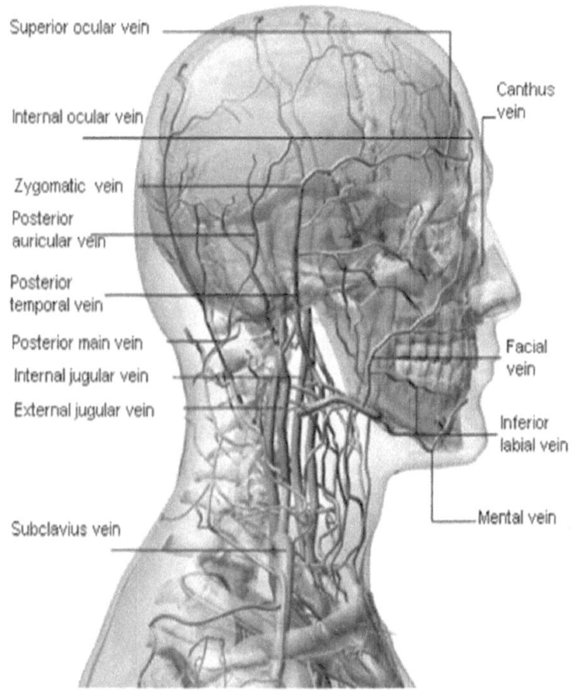

Unfortunately Royal Rife was ravaged by the FDA, his Lab was destroyed, and they attempted to eradicate his work. However it did exist, it did survive, he did develop a blue ray tube with a variable frequency modulator that changed frequencies according to each problem, disease, or whatever and he was able to cure them all. He did this in 1935-1938. And his work in America and pretty much in the world started this whole process. **Actually, the whole concept of inducing electrical signals into the body for healing purposes was first proposed by Nikola Tesla in 1888. He was the famous scientist that developed AC current generators in use today, as well as a large TENS unit which one would stand on and get stimulation through their feet. He used it daily, and died an old man in 1943.** However the real work came to be accomplished, and I say real work meaning the public production and marketing and information clinical studies put out which started in 1978 in Russia and 1979 in America. In Russia, work began on the SCENAR. The Russian scientists felt there was something we could do with this following what I said prior to this part, and so they started working on this concept. And in Russia they needed to have a small device that would replace hundreds of pounds of medical equipment because they couldn't fit all that stuff on Sputnik or the rocket ships they were developing. As we know the Russians were the first into space and so they were working on a space program using a small electrical device that could do all this work and they could carry into space.

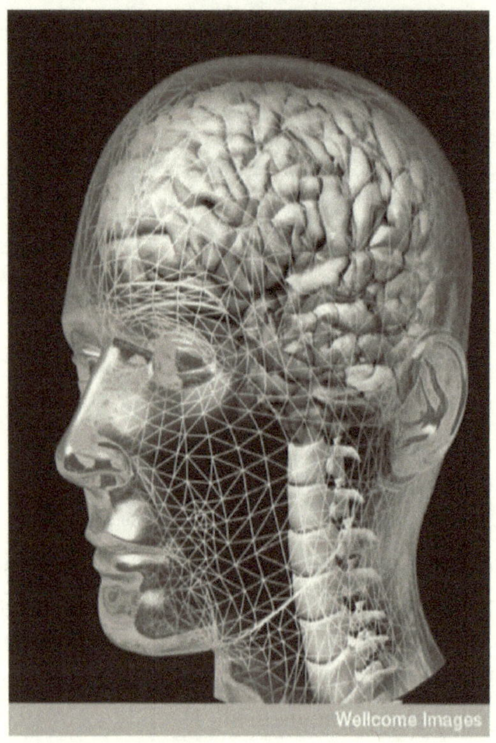

Meanwhile in America at a similar time, there was a bright young graduate student who was finishing his doctorate in Europe. He was contacted after returning to America by the founder of **Medtronic** and he was asked if he could invent a medical device that would stop the pain signal to the brain. And this bright young graduate student said, "Well certainly I can!" and he said "well come to work for us in Minnesota at Medtronic," and he did. And I did.

So he put me together with three other guys and we all started work on developing a small electronic device with the sole purpose of blocking the pain signal from the point of injury to the brain through the C fibers. Based on some work this fine young graduate student did on a previous experience at **McGill University** in Canada when he worked with **Dr. Ronald Melzack**, one of the co-discoverers of the gate control theory of pain, along with **Dr. Patrick Wall**. So the bright young graduate student, Dr. Wall and Dr. Melzack were nominated for a **Nobel Prize** for this work; however the bright young graduate student did not win the Nobel Prize because he, unlike his mentors at McGill University, did not write a textbook first.

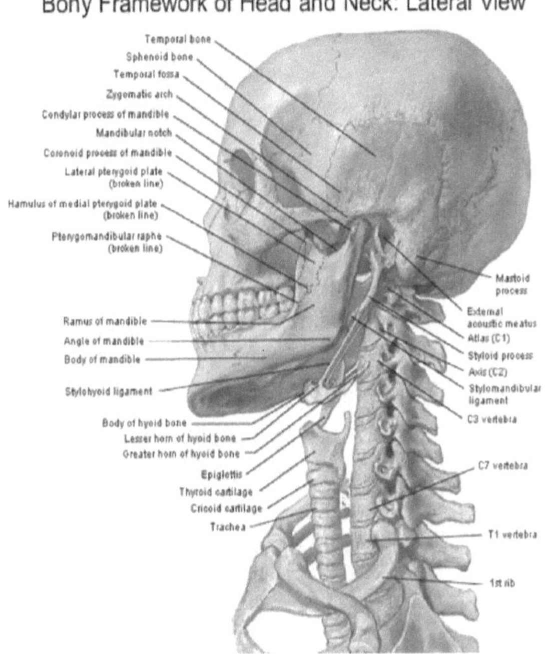

I went to Medtronic and we developed this small device and we put it out. It had two electrodes, it had a simple circuit inside and it put a conflicting signal into the body which stopped the pain signal and it was labeled a **TENS unit**. This device was co-invented by me, so I was not a bright young graduate student anymore. I got my first job out of graduate school. Not a bad start. We invented this device in America in 1980.

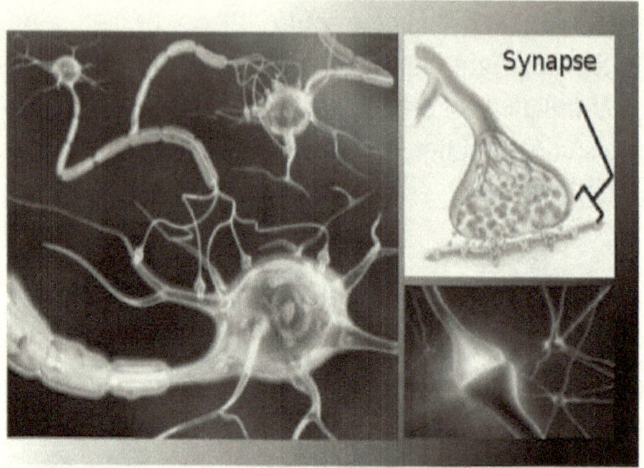

In the early phases of the Cosmonaut program, Russian scientists were grappling with the very real scenario of a health crisis in space. In that weightless environment, surgical procedures cannot be performed. Because of the confined areas of the space capsules and weight restrictions of the booster rockets, medicines and other health devices could not be taken along at the expense of oxygen, food, and waste disposal equipment. Large, heavy medical devices obviously could not be accommodated. **Pharmaceuticals** were totally impractical as well since they are designed to be so specific that a large pharmacy of many medications would be needed to cover even a few medical conditions. In addition, due to the limited supplies of potable water, all waste water must be recycled, which would concentrate medications into the drinking water and consequently treat all the personnel whether necessary or not.

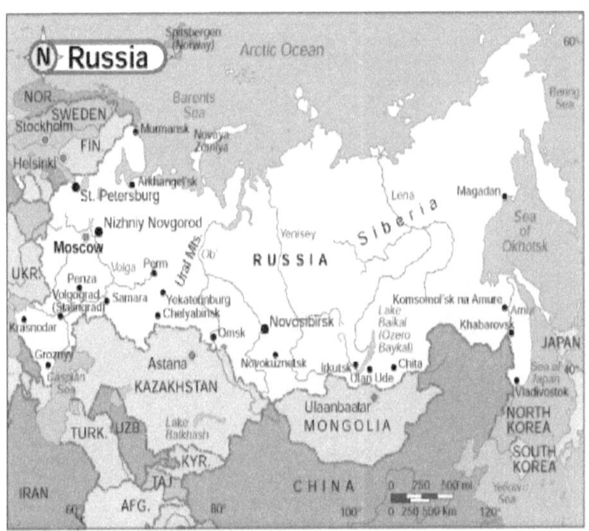

In the late 1970s the Russian Space Program established a special division to research and provide a resolution for this dilemma. This group was under the direction of electronics experts **Alexander Karasev** and **Alexander Nechushkin** as well as medical doctor and neurologist **Alexander Revenko.** They were headquartered at **Sochi University** and worked to develop an energetic medical device that could meet very exacting specifications. The device needed to be small and light enough to meet the size and weight restrictions of space flight, self-sufficient with a light power source, i.e., battery operated, be able to operate in the vacuum of space and capable of dealing with acute as well as chronic issues.

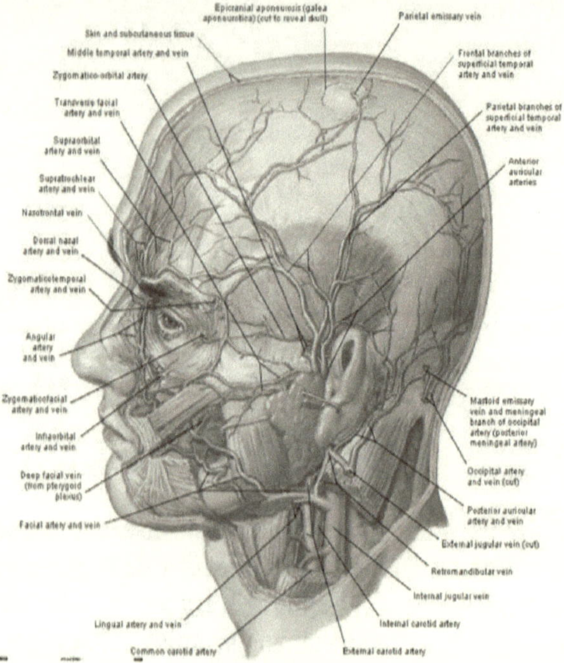

The end result of this program produced the **Scenar device**, or **Self-Controlled Energetic Neuro-Adaptive Regulator.** This device was kept as a highly classified military secret until the 1990s after Perestroika (the establishment of Gorbachev's policies of economic, political, and social restructuring and the breakup of the Soviet Union into its constituent republics). At that time the inventors received patents for the device and it was made available to western countries.

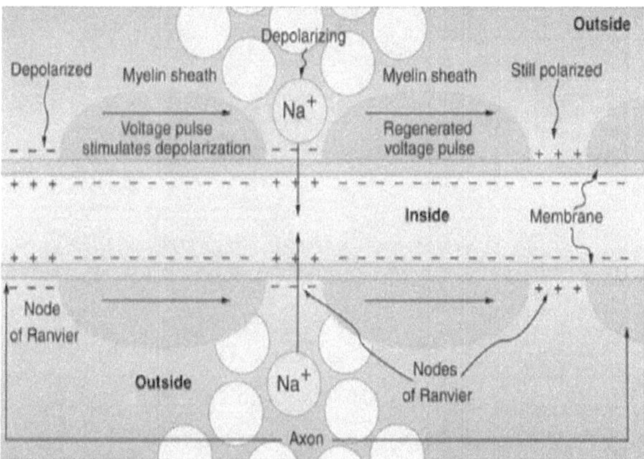

The **Scenar** received approval of the **USSR Medical Council** (Russia's FDA) in 1986 and was widely used in Russian hospitals. Many research papers have been published on its effectiveness. The inventors also received the Medal of Lenin (similar to a Nobel Prize) for its development.

From 1980 to this time the Russians and Americans are running and competing going forward with this technology. The now older Dr. Lathrop continued inventing medical devices all over the place that are still used today all over the country. There are names for them: **Electro-Accuscope, Myomatic, Mensomatic,** other **TENS units, Dynatron Lasers**, all these things were invented in America by the former bright young graduate student and in Russia there were two scientists who went about doing this as well. **Dr. A. Ravenko** and **Dr. A. Karasjev**. There were two scientists in Russia and two or three in America, namely Dr. Wing and Dr. Lathrop. So we had two pairs of scientists who were working furiously in two different countries to do this work. So we come now to the current time.

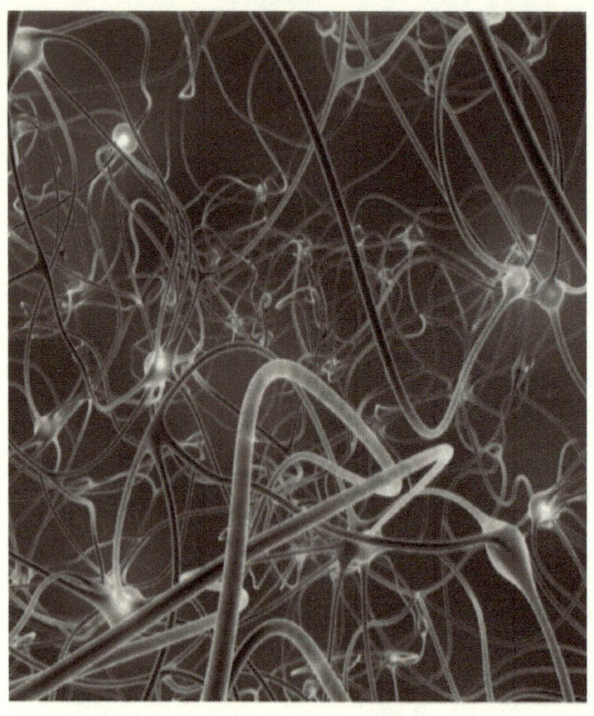

We have discovered that not only can we block pain, but we can also repair injuries following the concept/process described in my previous lecture. So we developed devices in America and in Russia. And as of today, 1980-2015, we now have devices that have been around for years, 10-15 years in America that are still considered 'new'! Why haven't I heard of that! Well they are not new. We have been doing this for years. I have been doing this for 35 years with these NEW amazing devices that no one has ever heard of.

They have been doing it in Russia the same way only they take it more seriously and the SCENAR is pretty much owned and used by every physician in Russia. In America not much. It's coming, it's growing, and it's getting to be known. This new amazing modern device - where has it been?

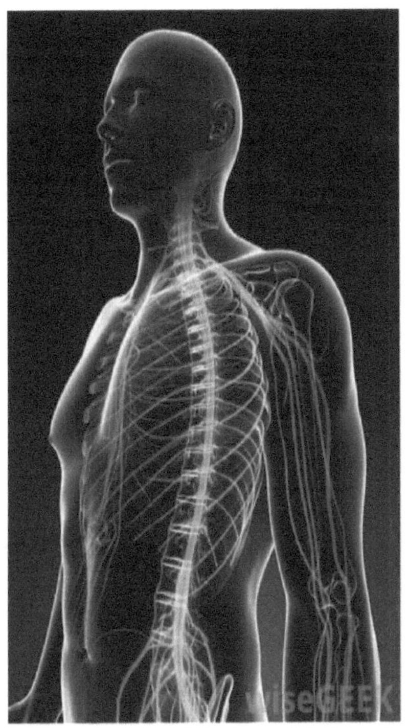

So now what we have is my inventions, which are pretty much big boxes with probes, as opposed to a hand held, remote control device which is SO usable, so convenient, which is so good and works so well, as well as anything I've invented if not better. So that's why we like it.

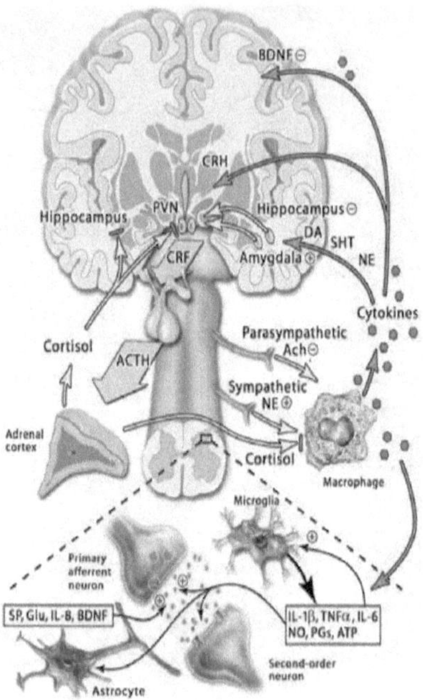

The point of it is, we now have a portable electronic device that will stop pain, repair injuries, correct internal medicine issues, repair internal organs and normalize the whole neurological system of the human body, if one wants to use it proactively and to keep their body healthy and never get diseases if you will. There are protocols for all of this, and we're doing it in clinical practice, laboratories and everywhere.